YOUR KNOWLEDGE HAS VALUE

- We will publish your bachelor's and master's thesis, essays and papers

- Your own eBook and book - sold worldwide in all relevant shops

- Earn money with each sale

Upload your text at www.GRIN.com and publish for free

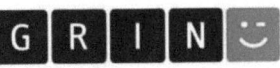

Uses of Fuel Efficient Stoves to improve Health Conditions of Women and Children in Ethiopia

Yohannes Asfaw Wakene

Bibliographic information published by the German National Library:

The German National Library lists this publication in the National Bibliography; detailed bibliographic data are available on the Internet at http://dnb.dnb.de.

ISBN: 9783346830166
This book is also available as an ebook.

© GRIN Publishing GmbH
Nymphenburger Straße 86
80636 München

Print and binding: Books on Demand GmbH, Norderstedt, Germany
Printed on acid-free paper from responsible sources.

The present work has been carefully prepared. Nevertheless, authors and publishers do not incur liability for the correctness of information, notes, links and advice as well as any printing errors.

GRIN web shop: https://www.grin.com/document/1334519

Table of Contents...I

ABRIVATION

AOR	Any Other Religion
CO$_2$	Carbon Dioxide
FES	Fuel Efficient Stove
FSS	Fuel Saving Stove
GHG	Green House Gas
HH	House Hold
FHHH	Female Headed House Hold
HOA	Horn of Africa
KAs	Kebele Administrations
LPG	Liquid Petroleum Gas
NGO	Non-Governmental Organization
OVC	Orphan and Vulnerable children
PFA	Primary Focus Area
SSA	Sub Saharan Africa
USEPA	Unite State Environmental Protection Agency.
USAID	United States Agency for International Development
UNDP	Unite Nation Development Program
WHO	World Health Organization
WVE	World Vision Ethiopia
WVA	World Vision Australia

ACKNOLEDGEMENT

Words do not express how great full to my Almighty God for always being with me and through my long education carrier. I would like to express my heartfelt gratitude to my advisor for reading the paper and making constrictive criticisms and valuable suggestion. Finally I would like to give credit to all who directly and indirectly involved in this research report writing in supporting me throughout my study.

ABSTRACT

Worldwide, 3 billion people are dependent on burning solid biomass fuels for cooking and heating needs (World Vision, 2011; Anhalt and Holanda, 2009; Sepp and Mann, 2009). Our country Ethiopia's rural people lack access to clean, affordable, and reliable energy and relay on traditional fuel use to meet their needs in this regards. In rural areas cooking is usually performed using traditional simple three-stone fire or "open fire". This traditional open firing consume much time and effort spent for gathering firewood and have adverse effect on households, particularly children and women wellbeing. Low-income communities located in rural areas without accesses to markets or energy infrastructures are most likely to benefit from improved cooking stove projects. However they are not benefiting. Hence, this research proposal aimed at divulging the role of fuel saving stove on the wellbeing of women and children in Lalo Assabi Woreda. These roles of improved stoves are: save energy, reduce the time and burden of collecting firewood, and limit the associated exposure for collectors to physical attack and/or gender based violence. To make this research real, a simple random techniques of primary data will be collect from 120 women/children under 15 years targets from three primary focus areas /PFA/, secondary data from line offices and NGO is mandatory.

1. INTRODUCTION

1.1. Background of the study

Many people are relying on wood fuel for cooking, lighting, and heating their home in countryside of Sub-Saharan African Countries in general and here in Ethiopia in particular. This has led to a significant burden for the planet and for those who are living on it. Unsustainable biomass collection depletes forests, contributes to soil erosion and loss of watersheds, placing additional pressure on agricultural productivity and food security which indirectly affect the living standards and well-being of human beings. At most searching for and using solid biomass fuels places women and children's safety at risk to human health and household and community air quality through toxic smoke emissions. In regions such as Sub-Saharan Africa countries /SSA/, where the lack of access to clean energy solutions and electrification is particularly significant, nearly a third of the urban population and the majority of the rural poor are using biomass for cooking and heating in traditional open fires that will affect their well-being in one way or the other. 2.5 billion people worldwide are fully dependent on burning biomass fuels for cooking. 1.6 million deaths each year mostly women and children can be attributed to diseases resulting from smoke inhalation from open cooking fires. Children are especially vulnerable to exposure from pollutants, which can impede the development of their organs and immune systems. Exposure to biomass smoke is a significant risk factor for acute lower respiratory infections in children, including pneumonia, which remains one of the most common causes of death in children under five globally. In developing countries, 730 million tons of biomass are burned each year, amounting to more than 1 billion tons of CO_2 in the atmosphere. Hence fuel efficient cooking stoves can reduce smoke inhalation with significant health benefits, save energy, reduce the time and burden of collecting firewood, and limit the associated exposure for collectors to physical attack and/or gender based violence by providing a host of social benefits.

1

1.2. Statement of the problem

This research report aimed at identifying the problem that women and girls/children encounter during collection of much biomass fire wood and face health risk at indoor activities when cooking. The research gives awareness for the community to use fuel saving stove that minimize fuel and reduce smoke that hazard their health. Many house hold from the district town and rural people knows nothing about fuel saving stove/FSS/ and are not using it in their home. They use traditional three stone fire or open fire for cooking, heating and lighting their houses. In a traditional open fire, three stones are placed in a triangular pattern on the ground, with the cooking pots resting on the stones directly above the fire. The open flame and lack of chimney or combustion chamber make this cooking fire inherently energy-inefficient. Rural women/ girls are consuming their time, energy their efforts in gathering fire wood from forest which is far from their home. As a result of this they don't have time for education, if they are student they don't have time for studying since they are responsible for role of cooking food in the household. When we compare boys with girl in the same house, girls role in household is much more tedious than the boy. Women/girls are exposed to sexual assault, rape, and kidnaps when they are going to collect firewood in the forest by men. As a result of this they are morally, physically and Psychologically harmed and their well-being will be affected.

On the other hand when women uses traditional three stone open fire by burning solid biomass fuels for cooking and heating, an indoor air pollution caused by traditional cooking stoves has great health threat, particularly for women and young children. Usually women/girls, spend several hours per day gathering fuel, increasing their daily labor and vulnerability to sexual violence While women and girls bear the brunt of clean energy poverty, their central and pivotal role in sustainable development is becoming increasingly clear.

In the area very few household are using different kinds of FSS. Very rarely institutions intervene for the existing problem. Therefore, this research will help show to provide information on the role of the FSS and the direction development planners to focus on the matter to save future generation not to be the victim of the mentioned problem.

Generally, this study was tried to answer the following question:

- ✓ How to identify the role of fuel efficient stove on the wellbeing of women and children in Lalo Assabi woreda?
- ✓ What are the relative advantages of FSS compared with traditional three stone stoves?

1.3. Research objective

General objective of the study:

- The general objective of the study is to identify the role of fuel efficient stove on the wellbeing of women and children at Lalo Assabi woreda.

The specific objectives of the study:

- To identify the relative advantages of FSS compared with traditional three stone stoves
- To recommend possible policy options that addresses the problem of fuel saving choice,

1.4. Significance of the study

Data on efficient cook stoves have been shown to result in significant social and economic benefits for adoptees and their families. The benefits fuel-efficient stoves are all rounded and cut across many development sectors, it is often hard to quantify or assign monetary value to these benefits, because many of them are indirect and fluctuate depending on a wide range of different factors. With a standard improved cook stove, for example, it will be possible to reduce cooking time and increase fuel efficiency. High efficiency cook stoves lead to even greater benefits in time and fuel savings and will significantly reduce harmful emissions. The additional time saved in fuel collection and cooking will result in more for women for work or to care for their families. Family who use improved stove will more likely to send their children to school. It also helps decreased drudgery, and improved health. The additional time saved will give ways to increased ability to pursue income generating or educational opportunities, and/or leisure activities and rest.

These all increase the awareness of the HH in Lalo Assabi Woreda regarding the role of fuel saving stove by providing the information for the HH. Likewise it recommend the possible policy options for the identified problem and help humanitarian organizations and government offices determine if an FES program is feasible and appropriate for a given setting of the area. Lastly, the study will be stepping stone in the area and will be a good input for future researchers to study the topic by including wider geographical area as well wider concepts.

1.5. Scope and limitations the study

Since the distance education learning was not easy to get clear ideas and instruction from the instructor/adviser being in distant in this course of action for this study. Yet I was not developed the skill of research work, there had been short comings on the process and practical investigations of my study. Likewise there has no access for internet to use except using phone internet. There was shortage of information from NGO and government office from the surrounding due to busy engagement in their activities to help show or involve in providing necessary secondary data information. There was no enough data concerning this topic even the available data was not properly put. Finally, financial and time constraints are also another limitation of this study.

2. LITERATURE REVIEW
2.1. Theoretical review

Worldwide, 3 billion people are dependent on burning biomass fuels for cooking (World Vision, 2011; Anhalt and Holanda, 2009; Sepp and Mann, 2009). In Sub-Saharan Africa (SSA), wood-based biomass is the dominant source of energy where about 81% of rural households and 60% of urban dwellers depend on it for cooking-far more than in any other region in the world (Modi et al., 2006; IBRD, 2011; World Vision, 2011 and Ekouevi and Tuntivate, 2012). Given current trends of population growth, urbanization, economic growth, and relative price developments of other energy sources, it is likely that wood-based biomass will remain an important source of energy for the coming many decades. Over 95% of the population in countries such as Burundi, Central African Republic, Chad, Liberia, Rwanda, The Gambia and Sierra Leone lack access to modern energy, with the rural population relying almost exclusively on wood based biomass energy for cooking. Wood-based biomass as the main source of energy is reported at 68% in Kenya, 95% in Eritrea, 94% in Ethiopia, while Zambia and Uganda indicated 70% and 92%, respectively

(Duflo and Greenstone, 2008 and UNDP, 2009 as cited by IBRD, 2011). Projections suggest that the consumption of wood-based biomass by SSA households will increase in relative terms over the next 30 years as demographic growth continues to outstrip access to other modern fuels (IBRD, 2011). Efforts to improve the efficiency of biomass cooking stoves date back to the 1940s. In recent decades, urban areas in developing nations have experienced higher dissemination rates of improved stoves; indeed, many urban households have made the switch to cleaner fuels like liquid petroleum gas (LPG) or kerosene for cooking. On the contrary, most rural households in these countries are not endowed with the necessary infrastructure that could bring them cleaner fuels, nor do they have the adequate income to pay for the fuels. Low-income communities located in rural areas without accesses to markets or energy infrastructures are most likely to benefit from improved cooking stove projects.((Duflo and Greenstone, 2008 and UNDP, 2009 as cited by IBRD, 2011).

One of the most powerful women in the world has talked about cooking stoves. She was Hillary Clinton and she described the huge impact that something as simple as cooking fuel has on millions of lives. This was one of the leading causes of death for women and small children. You might imagine HIV/Aids or, given the focus on maternal mortality at the UN Summit in New York, you might suggest that women's greatest risk is death in childbirth. But just as dangerous and much less well publicized is the risk of inhaling smoke from cooking on open fires which leads to lung and heart diseases. According to the United Nations, smoke costs 1.9 million lives a year.

Think about it; every day, millions of women across Africa and India spend several hours crouched over small fires cooking. Often their homes have no chimneys and poor ventilation. This daily proximity destroys lungs. Small children staying close to their mothers are equally vulnerable. Finally, this huge story is percolating through to the mainstream. Clinton is due to announce $50m (£32m) in seed money to the Global Alliance for Clean Cookstoves, to supply 100m fuel-efficient stoves across Africa.

Clean, sustainable energy supplies are going to become a crisis issue across eastern Africa. The pace of deforestation and population growth is such that experts predict that within 25 years, supplies of firewood – the main source of cooking fuel – will have largely run out. Given that the staple foodstuffs of these African countries require cooking (for example millet, sorghum), the impact on nutrition and hunger will be huge. And fuel impacts on women's lives in other ways; as the supplies become more scarce, they have to walk further and further to collect what they need, as the collecting of firewood is a woman's task. In places of conflict such as Darfur or Congo, it is collecting firewood which exposes women and children to the risk of rape.

This is a problem that does not require expensive technology. It is about using fuel efficiently.. We know exactly how to make these stoves at relatively low cost. The challenge is to distribute them fast enough to pre-empt the kind of crisis predicted for east Africa. One really interesting possibility is linking clean stoves to microfinance schemes enabling small local businesses to develop who will be able to sell the stoves.(Source: Clinton Alliance for Safe Motherhood.)

2.1.1 Definition of Stove

The term 'stove' refers to a device that generates heat from an energy carrier and makes that heat available for the intended use in a specific application. Cook stoves are made to transfer the generated heat to food, with the purpose to get it cooked and edible for human consumption. Thus 'a stove' features the combination of heat generation and heat transfer to a cooking pot if the food is cooked in a liquid, or a griddle, etc. if the food is baked on a hot surface or roasted without liquid.

2.1.2 Types of cooking stove

Cook stoves generally fall into two categories: Traditional and Improved cooking stoves

Traditional cooking stove

In traditional open fire, three stones are placed in a triangular pattern on the ground, with the cooking pots resting on the stones directly above the fire. The open flame and lack of chimney or combustion chamber make this cooking fire inherently energy-inefficient. Traditional stoves tend to be made of locally obtained materials such as stones or stones plus clay soil. Typically they are non-portable and built in situ by the user, who generally has little or no training in stove design and production. The dominant traditional cooking technology in developing countries is the "three-stone fire." This is one of the simplest cooking methods and is highly adaptable as it can utilize many types of fuel (i.e., firewood, crop residues, dung, leaves) and any type or size of cooking pot (metal or clay, flat- or round-bottomed). The three-stone fire consists of a cooking pot resting upon three stones or bricks that surround an open flame. It is free to build, simple to use, and can serve various non-cooking functions (such as providing a social gathering point). However, depending upon the cook's skill, the three-stone fire may require a lot of fuel, generate a lot of smoke, and present considerable safety risks from fires or burns. These are serious concerns in IDP situations, where fuel wood is expensive relative to the very low incomes, respiratory illness is common, and living quarters are both cramped and highly flammable. Most households in Darfur and in Sudan cook with both wood and charcoal. Many camp households use the traditional three-stone fire known locally as a ladaya, with all the attributes, both positive and negative, of this type of stove.

Respondents in the household survey were asked about their likes and dislikes concerning the three stone fire, and the responses are shown in Table 5.1. A vast majority of respondents thought that the three-stone fire used a lot of wood to cook a meal. Many respondents noted that it was a dangerous way to cook because the open flame could burn household members, especially children, and could cause fires in the straw huts that many households use as living quarters.

Household cooking energy is often discussed as a "one fuel - one stove" system. The archetype of this idea is the rural household using firewood in a 3-stone fireplace. On a second look, this picture is often a drastic simplification of the reality. Many households, particularly in (peri-) urban environments, are actually using several fuels and/or several stoves for a variety of reasons:

Different traditional meals require different types of heat (e.g. Ethiopia: the large pancake-style injera, sauce, and coffee ceremony);

Seasonal variation of availability or affordability of fuels (e.g. biomass as back-up if fossil fuels or electricity is not available, increasing prices or money shortages at the end of the month);

Variation of convenience needs (e.g. fast cooking in the morning, slow cooking in the evening);

Different abilities of cooks (e.g. expensive fuels and stoves shall not be used by the young daughter, so she is using firewood);

Different cooking needs (e.g. preparation of meals for the family on a different stove as the preparation of animal feed or processed food for the market);

Different types, shapes and sizes of cooking utensils (cooking pots, pans etc.) require different stove shapes or sizes.

Improved stove technologies

Fuel-efficient stoves are usually made with more sophisticated materials such as metal, fired bricks, or combinations of clay soil plus straw, cow dung, sawdust, or rice husks to improve insulation and durability. FES are often portable and some designs incorporate features for smoke removal. Some have complex design features and must be made by specialists, while others can be built by end-users themselves with appropriate training. Regardless of who makes the stove or where it is produced, users generally will need guidance to operate an FES properly and obtain the maximum benefits possible.

There are different types of improved stove found : (1) a simple mudstove, (2) an improved mud stove, (3) a six-brick Rocket stove /mirt, (4) a metal stove known as Tikikl stove, and (5) Lakech /charcoal burning stove.

Efficient stove: Cook stoves are commonly called "improved" if they are more "efficient" than the traditional cook stoves. But what does "efficient" mean in this case? Energy efficiency describes the heat transferred into the pot in relation to the overall energy generated by the stove within a defined task (e.g. water boiling test). But in most cases, this is not what is meant when the efficiency of stoves is discussed. From the perspective of a stove user, the core question concerning the efficiency of two alternative stoves is:

To use less fuel to prepare meal depends on the design stove that should considered the following factors:

- the quality of the fuel,
- Characteristics of the fuel,
- the handling of the fuel,
- the handling of the stove,
- the management of the cooking process and
- the cooking environment

When we talk about the efficiency of stoves, we usually compare the specific fuel consumption of a specific energy to either (a) a benchmark or (b) the specific consumption of another stove. Examples: Stove A consumes less fuel (for a specific standardized task) as indicated in the benchmark (e.g. 80g of charcoal per kg food prepared in a controlled cooking test) Stove A consumes 40% less fuel than stove B per litre boiled water (in a 5l Water boiling test)

A clay stove is perceived as an efficient stove in households with open fire places and as an inefficient stove in households which are using a rocket stove. International standards on stove quality have been discussed for many years. While they are desirable to enable a global comparison of stove performances, there is a danger that cheap solutions for the very poor households are abandoned due to their low performance in relation to the global standards, when in fact they could still be a relevant improvement in comparison to the baseline situation of the poorest of the poor. That's why a stratification of quality standards has been developed in the Lima consensus. Improved biomass cook stoves are thus to be considered a fuel-efficiency technology rather than a renewable energy production technology. Nevertheless, they are clearly a form of rural renewable energy use, one with enormous scope and consequences of use. Cook stoves come in a variety of designs targeting various types of biomass and cooking techniques that take into consideration cultural diversities. Improved stoves have been produced and commercialized to the largest extent in China and India, where governments have promoted their use, and in Kenya, where a large commercial market developed.

Global Stove Diversity

There are many different types of stoves across the world. This is natural, as a stove needs to accommodate the site-specific constellation determined by the available fuels, climatic conditions and preferences of users in the local culture. Thus, stove designs reflect global diversity. Please keep in mind: 'One size fits some, but rarely all'. The resulting diversity of stoves can be described in different categories such as:

Fuel types (solid, liquid or gaseous fuels from renewable biomass or fossil sources) Pot sizes (from small to big individual households sizes, medium to large pots for restaurants, enterprises or social institutions)

Stove designs also depend on the cooking habits. For instance, in many Latin American countries, tortillas are a traditional staple food baked on a hot metal plate ('plancha'). In Ethiopia the staple food is a pancake baked on a large ceramic plate. Stoves need to incorporate these essential features for people to prepare their staple foods. Otherwise the stove will not be acceptable in that area. Not all stove types comply with criteria required to qualify as 'improved stoves'. Promising stove types that are performing well within the GIZ-supported project areas are presented in the Stove Fact Sheets published by GIZ HERA.

Applications and Efficiency: Stoves can be largely categorized into domestic and institutional categories. This determines the design, size and cost. Institutional stoves tend to be bigger, more robust and generally more expensive in comparison to domestic stoves. Improved biomass stoves save from 10–50% of biomass consumption for the same cooking service provided and can dramatically improve indoor air quality. Research, dissemination, and commercialization efforts over the past few decades have brought a range of improved charcoal—and now wood-burning—stoves into use. Many of these stove designs, as well as the programs and policies that have supported their commercialization, have been highly successful.

There are 220 million improved stoves now in use around the world, due to a variety of public programs and successful private markets over the past two decades. This number compares with the roughly 570 million households worldwide that depend on traditional biomass as their primary cooking fuel. China's 180 million existing improved stoves now represent about 95% of such households. India's 34 million improved stoves represent about 25% of such households. In Kenya, the Ceramic Jiko stove (KCJ) is found in more than half of all urban homes and roughly 16–20% of rural homes. About one-third of African countries have programs for improved biomass cook-stoves, although there are few specific policies in place. Non-governmental organizations and small enterprises continue to promote and market stoves as well.

Policies and programs to promote efficient stoves are designed to improve the health, economic, and resource impacts of an existing renewable energy use and thus closely linked to sustainable forestry and land management.

2.2. Empirical review

Most empirical studies were conducted by using different methodologies regarding the role of fuel saving stove on the well-being of women and children. For example research conducted by Asfaw Eshete on Role of fuel efficient stoves in achieving the millennium development goals: case of Ethiopia mostly focus on women and children. Traditional fuel source have adverse effect on the environment, health, and economic development of people. The dominant source of traditional biomass energy is wood fuel/ fire wood and charcoal and the heavy reliance of traditional biomass is highly concentrated in rural areas were more than 90% of the population depends on this fuel (Alemu and Kaholin, 2008). The major part of SSA country fire wood is the most frequently cooking fuel. The performance of firewood on the energy economy of Africa follows both from its availability and its immediate low cost to the individual as well as it can be collected freely in the rural areas. The impact of traditional fuel on women and girl child will be more serious. They are affected by impact of using traditional fuel since women are responsible for collection, transportation, processing and storing, and as well as cooking activity in Ethiopia (Boris 2010).

3. RESEARCH METHODLOGY

3.1. Description of the Study Area

Lalo Asabi district is found in Western Wollega zone, about 464 Kms to the west of Addis Ababa, capital of the country. The total geographical area of the Woreda is 477km square with a total of 30 KAs (three of them are urban). The altitude of the district ranges from 1500 – 1800 m.a.s.l (meter above sea level) and the major agro-ecological zone of the area is Woina Dega having average annual precipitation ranging from 2043mm. As far as agro ecology of the area is concerned, the district is characterized by 100% mid land. Based on the recent census data the total population of the woreda is about 83,266 (43,536 male and 39,730 female).

The social and political situation of Lalo Assabi woreda is known to be steady and conducive. However, economic condition particularly the income of households is showing progress because of the effort of government and the intervention NGOs like WVE. The support of micro finances like WISDOM micro finance and Oromiya credit and saving institution are playing their part for improved economic situation. Government is doing a great work in constructing all weather roads in the district connecting Kebele to Kebele and with the neighboring districts that has paramount importance for increased communities' market access. In addition, job opportunities were created for number of community member by the WVE effort in off-farm income schemes and government small and micro enterprise policy. Infrastructures like electric power (in three town of the woreda) and telecommunication especially and mobile phone access is in continuous progress. In addition to WVE intervention, growth and transformation plan of the government is aggressively implanting has played significant role to rapidly growing social services such as health and education. These positive changes in turn support the progress of the program and its sustainability. Even though these all efforts were adopted in the district wood fuels are the most common sources of energy for the majority of the population in the district of Lalo Assabi. Firewood collection is often referred to as traditional fuels, yet they remain the dominant source of energy for cooking within the domestic sector, and are used extensively by all HHs. No any other access be found to fill their need in this regard like for instance electrification, and usage LPG …etc.

Furthermore they are unable to use improved fuel that minimize burden of fire wood collection from forest that expose them to many related problems except some town HHs.

3.2. Research Design

The researcher used descriptive type to use quantitative and qualitative research approach. Because command data collection and analysis method appeared consecutively with interview and questionnaire ,tables and percentages are used as well. This was expressed in terms of quantitative and qualitative research.

3.3. Source and Method of Data Collection

In this research primary data were collected from 121 sample HHs by using both open ended and closed ended questionnaires. The questionnaires were presented using face to face interview methods to the 121 respondents. Observation both traditional and improved stoves in respondent houses were included to augment the results from primary data. The researcher conducted survey to obtain primary, through interview and questionnaire and the secondary data was collected from books, journals and line offices.

3.4. Sampling Technique and Sampling Procedures

In order to obtain relevant and reliable data ,random sampling technique was used. Because random sampling technique is used to save time ,cost and gives equal chance for respondents. 121 HHs respondents were contacted for the study because of budget and time constraints out of the total 1200 people/population from three KAs . Priority will be given to women and girls in household during the random sample techniques at each KAs as we believe that culturally women are responsible for cooking activities in Ethiopia that made them only the victims of many problem. For this reason they rather than men are the focal area of the research study. There are women in Enango town and very few HH who are using FSS introduced by WVE and HOA and the stoves type is called "Mirti", "Tikikil", "Lakech" and mud stove.

3.4.1. Sample Size

For sorting out the impact of assessment of FSS on the wellbeing of women/girls, the researcher selected 121 sample from 1200 people by using the following formula

$$n = \frac{N}{1+N(e)^2}$$ where, n=sample size

N=total population

e= level of significance or acceptable error or level of precision.

Therefore, N=1200, e=8.6%,

$$n = \frac{1200}{1+1200(0.86)^2} == \frac{1200}{1+1200(0.007396)} == \frac{1200}{9.8752} = 121$$ sample size for the respondents were selected

3.5. Method of Data Analysis

The analytical tools employed for analysis were qualitative information, tabular and categorization method will be used as method of data analysis. For quantitative data, descriptive statics and regression model with different functional form will be used to analyze the data. A description and explanation of the elements, variables or factors to be measured or otherwise will be addressed.

4. RESULTSAND DISCUSSION

To undertake the study, the student researcher have to collect a primary data from respondents through questionnaires and interview. The researcher by assuming that sampling and presenting the opinion of respondents are relevant to the study. For the purpose of data analysis various variables are taken to account, which are used for sound and reliable information to users. The users and nonusers of FSS population has 1200 people three primary focus area, among these 121 respondents were selected as sample and the analyzed and presented as follows.

Table 4.1 The age distribution and total number of respondents

Number of respondents		
Age	Female	Percentage
10 - 18	15	12.40 %
19-28	40	33.06 %
29-35	50	41.32 %
>36	16	13.22 %
Total	121	100 %

Sources: Own survey 2016

From the above table of age category, we can understand that, from the total sample respondents 90 interviewees' age categories /the majority/ were between 19-35 ages and the remaining 31 interviewees' age categories /the youngest and the oldest/ were between 10-18 and above 36 ages. This shows that the majority of the women engaged in cooking processes were fall between 19-35 ages and they are the middle and productive age women.

Table 4.2 Respondents Religion

Religion	Number of respondents		percentage
	Female	**Total**	
Protestant	47	47	**39 %**
Orthodox	23	23	**19 %**
Catholic	0	0	**0 %**
Advents	42	42	**35 %**
Muslim	9	9	**7 %**
AOR	0	0	**0 %**
Total	121	121	**100 %**

Sources: Own survey 2016

From the above table the religion division of the respondents, we able to understand that from the total sample the majority of respondents, 39% percent were protestant, 35% percent belongs to advents and 19% percent were orthodox denomination followers. However the minority 7 percent religion division were Muslim. This shows that the majority of the women engaged in cooking processes fall in protestant and Adventist religion. Their religion category doesn't show any difference in the process of cooking. No support were pledged towards having this improved cooking stove for their members.

Table 4 .3. Educational level of respondents

Level of education	Number of respondents	Percentage
Uneducated	10	8.30 %
Primary school	54	44.60 %
Secondary school	46	38 %
College or University Graduate	11	9.10 %
Total	121	100 %

Sources: Own survey 2016

17

From the above 4. 3 table the large number of respondents have an educational status of primary school who were 54 in number or 44 % in percentage of the total respondents and the next large respondents have secondary school women who were 46 % in number or 38 in percentage and the remaining uneducated and college or university graduate that belongs to 10 and 11 in number and 8.3 % and 9.10 % in percentage respectively. This data shows that higher population of the respondents women were in primary and secondary school and the vice versa for uneducated and college or university graduates. The last minor educated of college or university graduate were the users of fuel efficient stove and are quick learner of the advantage of this better technology.

Table 4.4 Occupation of Head of the HH

Type of Occupation	Number of respondents	Percentage
Employed	5	4.13 %
Self employed	14	11.57 %
Housewife	102	84.30 %
Total	121	100 %

Sources: Own survey 2016

From the above 4.4 table, we can realize from the total respondents 5 of them or 4.13 % percent of the respondents were employed and were hired by government from the total respondents. Similarly, we can infer that the second minority 11.57 % or 14 respondents were self-employed or farmers and some of them were Female Headed Households /FHHH/. The majority 84.30 % percent or 102 respondents were housewife and are headed by husband and engaged in reproductive house role that incorporate all cooking process system, care for children and house hold management. This shows that almost all the respondents depends on self-employment and involved in the last mentioned house role activities.

Table 4 .5 Responsible person for cooking in the family

Responsible person	Number of respondents	Percentage
Adult man	0	0 %
Adult Woman	116	95.87 %
Female child under 18	5	4.13 %
Male child under 15	0	0 %
Others specify	0	0 %
Total	121	100 %

Sources: Own survey 2016

The above 4.5 table shows that, from the total sample of respondents 121, 95.87% percent of them /116 respondents/ are adult Woman and have responsibility for cooking in the family and the remaining 4.13% were female children under 18 ages /5 respondents in number/ and they were those whose mothers are sick and or OVC. From this data it could be possible to conclude that all in all women are responsible for cooking and heating in the house. In the rural area of Lalo Assabi cooking is accepted that it is the role and responsibility of women and no male engaged in cooking process. Rarely men and boys involved in the process if women posed to disease and no other girls found in that household. Men who engage in cooking process will be taken as inferior or rejected will have less value in front of other people.

Table 4 .6 Type of cooking fuel in the family

Types of fuel used	Number of respondents	Percentage
Electricity	0	0 %
Kerosene	5	4.13 %
Charcoal	10	8.30 %
Firewood	106	87.60 %
Total	121	100 %

Sources: Own survey 2016

The above table depict that, from the total sample respondents of 121, 87.60% of them are using firewood for cooking and heating purpose. The remaining 8.3% and 4.13% are rarely and interchangeably using charcoal and Kerosene respectively with biomass collected fuel to minimize cost of purchasing kerosene and charcoal. In addition there are no respondents who are using electricity as a source of fuel for cooking and heating their home. This shows that majority of the respondents in the study area depends on firewood for cooking traditionally on three stone open fire.

Table 4 .7 Type of cooking stove used in the family

Types of stove the respondent use	Number of respondents	Percentage
Tikikil	10	8.30
Mirt	19	15.70
Mud stove	23	19
Non stove users	69	57.03
Total	121	100

Sources: Own survey 2016

From the above 4.7 table, we can understand that, from the total sample respondents of 121, 57% of them /69 respondents/ are not using fuel efficient stove. The remaining 19%, 15.70% and 8.30% are using different kinds of cooking stove respectively. This indicate that majority of the respondents were non users of fuel efficient stoves and using traditional three stone open fires.

Table 4 .8 Condition and security of roads in the forest

Condition of roads	Number of respondents	Percentage
Safest	0	0 %
Safe	12	9.92 %
Not safe	48	39.67 %
Worst	61	50.41 %
Total	121	100 %

Sources: Own survey 2016

From the above table, we can understand that, from the total sample respondents of 121, 50.41% and 39.67% of them are explained the situations of the road are worst and not safe. In line with this from the total respondents 9.92% feel safe to the condition of the roads to collection of firewood. This indicate that majority of the respondents were not feel good to the situation of road when collecting fire wood and some are victims sexual of assault though don't need to disclose the risks to the interviewers.

Table 4 .9 Frequency of gathering fire wood from forest

Frequency	Number of respondents	Percentage
Once in two weeks	15	12.40 %
Once in a week	39	32.23 %
Twice in a week	52	42.98 %
Triple in a week	15	12.40 %
Total	121	100

Sources: Own survey 2016

From the above table, we can understand that, from the total sample respondents of 121, the majority or 43% and 32.30% collect firewood twice and once in a week for cooking respectively. The remaining 12.40% of the total respondents are collecting firewood once in two weeks and triple in a week respectively. Those who are collecting fire woods once in two weeks are those who are using kerosene and charcoal interchangeably with firewood and those who collect firewood triple in a week are women who are engaged in business interlinked with cooking like backing injera or bread and also producing katukala or what we call alcohol production. This indicate that majority of the respondents were non users of fuel efficient stoves and using traditional three stone open fires that uses fuel inefficiently.

Table 4 .10 Role of fuel saving stove

Role of fuel saving stove in Lalo Assabi Woreda	Number of respondents know the role &responded (Yes)	Number of respondents who don't know the role and responded (No)	Rank
1. Helps to reduce smokes	93	28	1st
2. Keep cleanliness of the kitchen/house	90	31	3rd
3. Keep children from burnt	88	33	4th
4. Help reduce the frequency of fire wood collection	86	35	5th
5. Contribute to education for women/girls	84	37	6th
6. Help women to involve in income generation interventions	83	38	7th
7. Reduce respiratory/lung and eye illness	91	30	2nd
8. Help to reduce sexual assault to women	82	39	8th
9. Contribute to other social benefit	81	40	9th

Source: Own survey 2016

Out of the sample respondents, 57% of them were totally not using fuel efficient stove and they are using traditional three stone open fire. From the above table in average 28% of them did not know the role of improved stove versus the traditional one. In line with this 29% of them were not using this stove however they identify the role that FSS have over that of traditional one and responded positively. The remaining 43% use improved stove interchangeably with that of traditional one. There are respondents who use portable stove called Lakech in local language that help them only for boiling of coffee/tea and rarely for cooking stew otherwise they use traditional stove for cooking big meal and they are estimated to be 20% and the remaining 23% use FSS.

According to the above result findings 77% (93 respondents), 75% (91 respondents) and 74% (90 respondents)prioritize the role of stove "helps to reduce smoke", "reduces respiratory and eye illness" and " keep cleanliness of the kitchen" respectively. The respondents mentioned that traditional cooking have problem much smoke that made their eye to become ill and lead to blindness in the long run. This smoke inhalation for long time can cause, coughing, common cold, headache and asthma. In addition constantly cooking with traditional stove can bring back pain as a result it can cause back disc dislocation. Hence, majority of women in the countryside suffer from mentioned problem as the respondents replied and improved stove users that the mentioned problem were minimized in their house. "Keep children from burnt" role of fuel saving stove rank stood 4th. Depending on the results obtained from respondents as children in their home were especially vulnerable burnt since they spend much time indoors close to their mothers who are cooking.

Similarly the results of the respondents shows 71% (86 respondents), 69% (84 respondents) and 70% (83 respondents) prioritize accordingly for the role of FSS "help reduce the frequency of fire wood collection, "contribute to education for women" and "help women to involve in income generation interventions" respectively. As respondents replied towards the mentioned 5th, 6th and 7th rank specially improved stove made of mud stove, tikikil, and mirt with chimney have no smoke and consume less fuel when compared with that of traditional one. As a result frequency collection of biomass from forest reduced that can contribute for women to have ample time for education/studying and income generating activities. 43% of respondent who use FSS have their girls at school and the women were engaged in petty trading and home guarding activity and their living standard on the process of improving. Role of FSS called " help to reduce sexual attack" and "contribute to other social benefits" were prioritized the last 8th and 9th compared to other roles. The contribution of improved stove towards these roles were not minimal that make it stood last however it was relatively that they saw. The respondents did not disclose themselves towards the effect of sexual attack but there are   women/girls in the area who are the victims of the problem.

The victims are morally, physically and psychologically harmed and their well-being were affected, that they did not get married and women who married were disagreed by their spouse and prone to divorce.

With regards to the role of fuel saving stove previous research findings, no prioritization and ranking were made but only qualitative description were made. There were increasing evidence that the burning of solid biomass fuels for cooking in indoor mainly using traditional stoves in inadequately ventilated spaces, can lead to an increased disease burden for the cooker and burnt of children in the fire. Cooking and heating with solid fuels on open fires or on traditional stoves generates high levels of health damaging pollutants, indoor air pollution is a major contributing factor for ill health in rural communities due to inefficient burning of fuel wood, along with poor ventilation systems inside houses (Asfaw Eshete's research on the role of fuel saving stove in achieving MDG)

According to the World Vision international reports traditional three stone open fire users view; Women, children and older persons, who spend most of their time indoors, are severely affected. Women who are engaged in cooking and heating with traditional stove for a long time have daily discomfort from coughs, headaches, stinging of eyes and backaches were some of the critical health problems associated with exposure to indoor air pollution.

Girls are consuming their time, energy, their efforts in gathering fire wood from forest which is far from their home triple and twice a week from long distance for the scarcity of biomass fuel and as a result they don't have time for education, if they are student they don't have time for studying since they are responsible for role of cooking heating house in the household. Boys and girls were compared in the same house and girls role in household is much more tedious than the boy she engaged more in fulfilling processes heating and cooking meals for the member of the household but not doing business of her own education, a major reason for keeping girls aged 10 to 12 out of school is to help the mothers collect firewood. There were Women/girls who are encountered sexual assault, rape, and kidnaps and they are vulnerability also to cuts, animal bites, falls as they travel long distances during going and coming to and from collection of firewood in the forest by men.

FSS utilization enables them more time for female students to attend school, Health status improved for them and their children Increase labor productivity as Wood collection time reduced, Minimize indoor air pollution, Fuel wood demand reduced for their daily cooking activities. Any reduction in pollutants emitted from cook stoves will be beneficial for children's as well as for women's health. Cleaner fuels and cook stoves that facilitate lower smoke exposures, as well as improved ventilation of cooking areas, can reduce the disease burden from smoke, lower child mortality rates, and improve maternal health. Respondents with access to a reliable FSS and modern energy supply will free women and girls from this chore, providing time for activities such to engage in their education and income generation activities. When fuel efficient stoves are widely used, the disproportionate amount of daily time and effort women and young girls spend gathering solid fuels for household chores could be used for other income-producing activities,

Table 4 .11 Relative advantages of FSS with that of traditional one

Relative advantages of FSS compared with traditional three stone stoves Which one is better to		No. of respondents on the advantage of FSS	Relative advantage percentage of FSS	Total respondents
i.	Save cooking time	79	65	121
ii.	Reduce fuel	79	65	121
iii.	Reduced smoke	79	65	121
iv.	Accessible easily	93	78	121
v.	Affordable	79	65	121
vi.	Safest	91	77	121
vii.	Easier to use	80	66	121
viii.	Effective in cooking range of food at a time	91	77	121

Own survey 2016

From the total respondents on average 71% knows the relative advantage of FSS and 29% (36 respondents) of them doesn't identify and experience the relative advantage that improved fuel saving stove have. In other words out of the total respondents 85 women know and experience the relative advantage of the improved stove but 36 of them did not identify the relative advantage of the stove. Out of the non-users of (57%) only 27% knows the relative advantage of improved stove because they sow the process of stove functioning from their neighbors but could not afford buying for use because of economic capacity.

27

Specifically 79 respondents know the relative advantage "reduce cooking time, fuel, time, smoke and affordability". 91 respondents understand the advantage of safest and effective in cooking range of food at a time that FSS have over traditional stove. 80 of them found this stove easier to use than the open fire cooking.

According to the respondents saying FSS is Cleaner than three-stone, Less smoke, no fire burnt danger, its wood efficient, couldn't cause house fire and safer, its modern, easy to use, saves time, remains warm overnight, and Less supervision needed. From the above table FSS users know what improved stove mean for them however those who are using traditional one still have less know how about what the difference it has.

Table 4:12 Role and Relative advantage of FSS summary table

No	description	No. of respondents	Percentage	Remark
1	Non-users of FSS	69	57%	
2	Users of FSS	52	43%	
	Total	**121**	**100%**	
3	Know the relative advantage	85	71%	
4	Not know the relative advantage	36	29%	
	Total	**121**	**100%**	

N.B: From the non-users (69 respondents) 33 respondents (27%) understand the relative advantage of FSS but couldn't afford due to economic capacity.

Own analysis 2016

4. CONCLUSION AND RECOMMENDATION

4.1 Summary

Access to energy is a basic human need and have more challenge to rural people in improving their welfare. The vast majority people rely on traditional biomass collection for cooking, lighting and heating respectively, which can have significant negative impacts on their well-being. This is particularly true for women and children, who may be exposed to health and safety risks and have less time for education, livelihoods, social and other activities because of the time they spend in collecting fuel. Millions of deaths each year mostly women and children can be attributed to diseases resulting from smoke inhalation from open cooking fires. Children are especially vulnerable to exposure from pollutants, which can impede the development of their organs and immune systems. Exposure to biomass smoke is a significant risk factor for acute lower respiratory infections in children, including pneumonia, which remains one of the most common causes of death in children under five globally.

Hence, the benefits of introducing improved fuel-efficient stoves were all rounded and cut across many development sectors. It is often impossible to quantify or assign monetary value to those positive roles to our mothers and sisters. Therefore, it is imperative to give emphasis in identifying the associated problems to disseminating the role and advantage fuel saving stove has for the wellbeing of rural women and improves their living standards.

4.2 Conclusion

In this paper, the researcher tries to assess the role and advantage of fuel saving stove on the well-being of women and girls for the case of Lalo Assabi district. Based on the result of the respondents we can infer that the Majority of the district HH were engaged in using traditional open fire system for cooking, lighting and heating their home. In doing so they did not identify the role and the flipside stove have. It can help save energy, reduce the time and burden of collecting firewood, and limit the associated exposure for collectors to health risks, physical attack and/or gender based violence though they are experiencing the problem. Very few of them identify the benefits of improved fuel efficient stove and are using. They recognized improved stoves have several role towards the mentioned bottlenecks problem to their welfare that it reduces the amount of indoor air pollution in a home and, therefore, can improve a family's health. They become aware that it can reduce the money spent to purchase fuel (for women who are living in small town of the district) because they require less fuel than traditional stoves. Therefore, most of the benefits of having improved stoves involve in reducing the fuel collection time for household members, especially for women and give an opportunity to engage in studying and income generation activities. In general, improved cooking stoves increase cooking efficiency compared with a traditional stove; can reduce fuel gathering time, and cooking time all of which have the potential to improve health and increase household income thus increase the welfare of women and girls/children in rural areas.

4.3 Recommendations

In light of the conclusion the following recommendations are drawn in the hope that they would help to address the problem of the community of Lalo Assabi.

1. Even though there are some efforts done in the district to combat the effect of traditional open fire cooking system by the government and Humanitarian Non-Governmental Organizations so far, there are still many household who are not the beneficiaries of this clean energy technology. Therefore, the concerned bodies should work more towards in disseminating and publicizing appropriate fuel efficient technologies to the rural community in Lalo Assabi district areas to ensure the wellbeing of our mothers, wives, sisters and children in rural areas.

2. Since there are women in the area who are using this improved clean energy technology, and the provision is affordable for buying the stove, its mandatory for the district line offices as well zone office and NGO working there to mobilize and build the capacity of the community to have it in their home to earn the fruit of the technology.

3. Trying to call humanitarian organization to establishing local craftswomen and artesian women groups to support in stove mold, and train them for the production appropriate stove for the area for sale in the vicinity.

4. To share experience between users and non-users of FSS in the district to make rural women identify the role and advantage easily and differently.

REFERENCE

Alvarez D., C. Palma & M Tay (2004). Evaluation of Improved Stove Programs in Guatemala: Final report of project case studies. ESMAP Technical Paper 060.

Health Care Delivery in Rural Rajasthan. Economic and Political Weekly, 39 (9): 944-949.

Banres D & J. Halpern (2000). The Role of Energy Subsidies. In the World Bank's "Energy and Development Report 2000: Energy Services for the World's Poor."

Environmental Protection Agency (2006). Particulate Matter Standards. USEPA. Last accessed 1/9/07. WHO Energy for cooking in developing countries Helen 2005; Alemu and Kohlin 2008). Woreda Mine, energy and water office Report 2005 Zone Mine, energy and water office Report 2005 World Vision Ethiopia Area Program report 2009 WHO Factsheet (2014) http://www.who.int/mediacentre/factsheets/fs2 92/en/ WRC. (2011). Cooking fuel saves lives: Protection. Women's Refugee Commission (Duflo and Greenstone, 2008 and UNDP, 2009 as cited by IBRD, 2011).[1] UNCHR, Refugee Operations and Environmental Management, A Handbook of Selected Lessons Learned from the Field, 2002.

[1] Stephen Gitonga, "Energy Options for Refugee Camps," *Boiling Point* Issue 37, 1996.(Gill, 1985; FAO, 2003; UNDP, 2005b; Barnes et al., 2012 and Ekouevi and Tuntivate, 2012).

ANNEX 1

JIMMA UNIVERSITY

COLLEGE OF AGRICULTURE,

DEPARTMENT OF AGRICULTURAL ECONOMICS AND RURAL DEVELOPMENT

QUESTIONNAIRE

Questionnaire to be filled by users and non-users of Fuel Saving Stove of LaloAssabi district .

Part I. Socio-economic Questionnaire

1. What is your sex? A) Female B) Male
2. What is your age? _____
3. What is your marital status? A) Married B) Single C) Divorced D) Widowed
4. What is your religion? A) Orthodox B) Catholic C) Protestant D) Muslim E) Adventist F) AOR
5. What is the level of your education? A) Uneducated B) Primary school C) Secondary School D) College or University graduate
6. What is Occupation of Head of the HH in your family? A) Employed B) Unemployed

Part II Questionnaire on the role of FSS

The aim of this part is to identify role of FSS for women and children/girls.

7. Who is responsible for cooking activities in your family? A) Adult man B) Adult Woman C) Female child under 15 D) Male child under 15 E) Others specify_____
8. Which type of cooking fuel do you use frequently? A) Electricity B) Kerosene C) Charcoal D) Firewood
9. Are the roads in to/out of the forest during firewood collection safe to travel regularly?
10. How often do you go to gather your fuel per week? _____
11. If you engage in gathering fuel wood from forest do you experience problem in the process?

33

12. What kind of problem?_____

_____

13. What type of stoves are currently being used by the population?

    Type 1_____

    Type 2_____

    Type 3_____

    Type 4_____

14. Have you or another family member ever burned using this stove?_____

Role of fuel saving stove in Lalo Asabi Woreda	Yes	No
a. Helps to reduce smokes		
b. Keep cleanliness of the kitchen/house		
c. Keep children from burnt		
d. Help reduce the frequency of fire wood collection		
e. Contribute to education for women/girls		

f. Contribute to other social benefit		

Part III. Questionnaire on challenges of micro and small scale enterprise for urban poor household

Relative advantages of FSS compared with traditional three stone stoves Which one is better to	FSS	Traditional three stone stoves (Open fire)
i. Save cooking time		
ii. Reduce fuel		
iii. Reduced smoke		
iv. Accessible easily		
v. Affordable		
vi. Safest		
vii. Easier to use		
viii. Effective in cooking range of food at a time		
ix. Large quantity cooking		

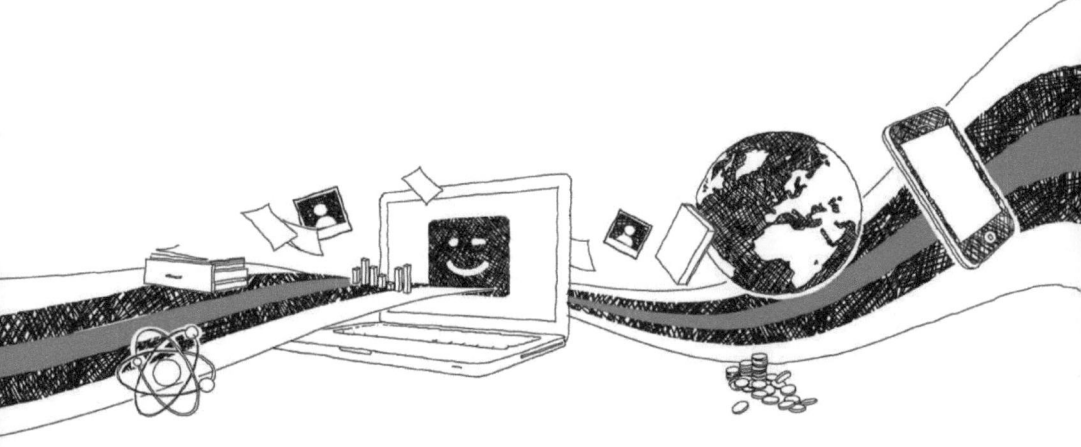
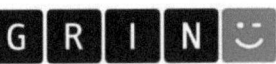